The Healing Power of Augmented Reality
Revolutionizing Medicine

Oakley Sean

Copyright © [2023]

Title: The Healing Power of Augmented Reality Revolutionizing Medicine
Author's: Oakley Sean

This book was printed and published by [Publisher's: **Oakley Sean**]   in [2023]

ISBN:

TABLE OF CONTENT

Chapter 1: Introduction to Augmented Reality in Healthcare

The Emergence of Augmented Reality Technology

Overview of the Book's Purpose and Structure

Chapter 2: Understanding Augmented Reality

Definition and Explanation of Augmented Reality

Historical Development of Augmented Reality

Types of Augmented Reality Systems

Chapter 3: Augmented Reality in Medical Education and Training

Enhancing Medical Education with Augmented Reality

Virtual Anatomy Simulations

Surgical Training and Visualization

Patient Interaction and Communication

Benefits and Limitations of Augmented Reality in Medical Education

Chapter 6: Future Perspectives and Challenges   48

Advancements in Augmented Reality Technology

Integrating Augmented Reality into the Healthcare System

Overcoming Barriers to Implementation

Implications for Medical Research and Innovation

Chapter 7: Conclusion   57

Recap of Key Points

Chapter 1: Introduction to Augmented Reality in Healthcare

The Emergence of Augmented Reality Technology

In recent years, there has been a remarkable emergence of augmented reality technology, revolutionizing various industries and transforming the way we perceive and interact with the world around us. Augmented reality, often abbreviated as AR, is a cutting-edge technology that combines the real world with computer-generated virtual elements, enhancing our sensory experiences and opening up new possibilities in fields such as medicine, education, gaming, and more.

At its core, augmented reality technology overlays digital content onto our physical environment, seamlessly blending the two worlds together. This is made possible through the use of advanced sensors, cameras, and displays, which enable real-time tracking and rendering of virtual objects onto our screens or even directly onto our surroundings. The result is an immersive and interactive experience that has captivated the imagination of people across all walks of life.

One of the most exciting applications of augmented reality technology can be found in the field of medicine. Its potential to revolutionize healthcare is immense, as it allows medical professionals to visualize complex anatomical structures, such as organs and blood vessels, in a three-dimensional space. Surgeons can use AR during operations to overlay real-time patient data, such as vital signs and imaging scans, directly onto their field of view, enabling more precise and informed decision-making. Additionally, AR can be used in medical education, providing students with realistic simulations and interactive learning experiences that were previously unimaginable.

Beyond medicine, augmented reality has also found its way into the world of entertainment and gaming. With the advent of smartphone technology, anyone with a mobile device can now experience the thrill of augmented reality games. These games blend the real world with virtual elements, allowing players to interact with digital characters and objects in their own environment. From hunting virtual creatures in Pokémon GO to defending their living rooms from alien invasions, augmented reality gaming has captured the hearts of millions and continues to push the boundaries of what is possible in the gaming industry.

In conclusion, augmented reality technology has emerged as a powerful tool that is transforming various industries and captivating the imagination of people from all walks of life. Whether it is revolutionizing medicine by enhancing surgical procedures and medical education or providing immersive gaming experiences, augmented reality is reshaping the way we perceive and interact with the world around us. As this technology continues to evolve, the possibilities for its applications are virtually limitless, and it is bound to have a lasting impact on our daily lives.

Overview of the Book's Purpose and Structure

"The Healing Power of Augmented Reality: Revolutionizing Medicine" is a groundbreaking book that explores the immense potential of augmented reality (AR) in transforming the field of medicine. With its ability to overlay virtual elements on the real world, AR has the power to revolutionize healthcare, enhancing medical education, improving patient outcomes, and revolutionizing the way healthcare professionals deliver care.

This book is designed to provide an in-depth understanding of the healing power of augmented reality, catering to a wide range of readers, from healthcare professionals to technology enthusiasts. Whether you are a physician, a nurse, a medical student, a developer, or simply someone interested in the future of healthcare, this book will offer valuable insights into the world of AR and its implications for medicine.

The book begins with an introduction that sets the stage for the readers, explaining the concept of augmented reality and its relevance in the medical field. It delves into the history of AR, highlighting key breakthroughs and advancements that have led to its current state. This section aims to familiarize the audience with the fundamental concepts of AR, ensuring a solid foundation for the subsequent chapters.

The subsequent chapters explore the various applications of augmented reality in medicine. Each chapter focuses on a specific niche within the field of medicine, demonstrating how AR can be utilized to improve patient care, enhance medical training, and revolutionize diagnostics and treatment. From surgical simulations to telemedicine, from medical education to rehabilitation, each chapter offers practical examples and case studies that highlight the benefits of AR in real-world scenarios.

Throughout the book, the authors draw upon the expertise of leading professionals in the fields of medicine and technology. Interviews with renowned physicians, researchers, and developers provide valuable insights and perspectives, further enriching the reader's understanding of the subject matter.

The book concludes with a visionary outlook on the future of augmented reality in medicine. It explores the potential challenges and ethical considerations that may arise as AR becomes more integrated into healthcare systems. It also offers practical advice for individuals interested in pursuing a career in the intersection of medicine and augmented reality, providing resources and guidance to help readers embark on their own journey in this exciting field.

"The Healing Power of Augmented Reality: Revolutionizing Medicine" is a comprehensive guide that aims to inspire and educate readers about the transformative potential of AR in medicine. Whether you are a healthcare professional looking to enhance your practice or a technology enthusiast curious about the future of healthcare, this book will undoubtedly broaden your horizons and leave you excited about the possibilities that lie ahead.

Chapter 2: Understanding Augmented Reality

Definition and Explanation of Augmented Reality

Augmented Reality (AR) is a revolutionary technology that has the potential to transform various industries, including medicine. In simple terms, AR refers to the integration of digital information, such as graphics, sounds, and haptic feedback, into the real-world environment. Unlike virtual reality, which creates an entirely artificial world, AR enhances the real-world environment by overlaying digital content onto it.

Imagine wearing a pair of AR glasses and being able to see virtual objects, data, or even holograms seamlessly integrated into your surroundings. This technology has the power to provide real-time information, improve communication, and enhance our perception of the world around us. It offers endless possibilities, whether in education, entertainment, or healthcare.

In the context of medicine, augmented reality has the potential to revolutionize the way we diagnose, treat, and even prevent illnesses. By superimposing medical data onto a patient's body, doctors can gain a deeper understanding of complex anatomical structures, aiding in accurate diagnoses. Surgeons can also benefit from AR during procedures, as it allows them to visualize critical information, such as the location of blood vessels or nerves, in real-time.

One of the most significant advantages of AR in medicine is its ability to enhance medical training and education. Students and healthcare professionals can use AR to practice complex procedures, improve surgical skills, and gain hands-on experience in a safe and controlled environment. This technology bridges the gap between theory and practice, facilitating a more immersive and effective learning experience.

Furthermore, augmented reality can improve patient outcomes and experiences. With AR, doctors can create personalized treatment plans based on a patient's specific needs and conditions. Patients can also benefit from AR by visualizing their own health data, understanding their conditions better, and actively participating in their treatment journey.

As AR continues to evolve, its impact on medicine will only grow. From telemedicine to remote surgeries, the possibilities are endless. However, there are still challenges to overcome, such as privacy concerns and the need for seamless integration into existing healthcare systems. Nonetheless, the healing power of augmented reality is undeniable, and its potential to revolutionize medicine is awe-inspiring.

In conclusion, augmented reality is a groundbreaking technology that enhances our perception of reality by overlaying digital content onto the real-world environment. In medicine, AR has the potential to transform how we diagnose, treat, and educate. From improved diagnostics to enhanced surgical procedures, this technology offers endless possibilities for improving patient outcomes and experiences. Although challenges exist, the healing power of augmented reality is poised to revolutionize medicine and usher in a new era of healthcare.

Historical Development of Augmented Reality

Augmented Reality (AR) has emerged as a groundbreaking technology that has the potential to revolutionize various industries, including medicine. To truly understand the impact and potential of AR in healthcare, it is essential to explore its historical development and how it has evolved over time.

The roots of AR can be traced back to the 1960s when computer scientist Ivan Sutherland introduced the concept of a "head-mounted display" that could overlay computer-generated graphics onto the real world. This early work paved the way for subsequent advancements in the field of AR.

In the 1990s, the term "augmented reality" was coined by Tom Caudell, a researcher at Boeing, to describe a digital display system that assisted aircraft assembly workers. This marked a significant milestone in the development of AR, as it highlighted its potential to enhance real-world tasks with computer-generated information.

The early 2000s saw the emergence of AR applications in various industries, including entertainment and gaming. Companies like Nintendo popularized AR through their handheld gaming devices, allowing users to interact with virtual characters and objects in the real world.

However, it was not until the release of smartphones with built-in cameras and advanced computing capabilities that AR truly took off. In 2008, the first AR application for smartphones, called "Wikitude," was launched, allowing users to access location-based information by simply pointing their phone's camera at a specific area.

Since then, AR has continued to evolve, with major tech giants like Google and Apple investing heavily in the technology. Google's "Project Glass" and Apple's introduction of the ARKit framework have further pushed the boundaries of AR, making it more accessible and user-friendly.

In the field of medicine, AR has begun to play a significant role in surgical planning, training, and patient care. Surgeons can now use AR to overlay 3D models of a patient's anatomy onto their field of view, providing real-time guidance during complex procedures. AR also facilitates medical education by enabling students to visualize and interact with anatomical structures in ways previously unimaginable.

Looking ahead, the future of AR in medicine holds immense potential. From improving patient outcomes to revolutionizing medical education, AR is set to transform the healthcare landscape. As technology continues to advance, the possibilities for AR in medicine are limitless.

In conclusion, the historical development of augmented reality has been a journey of innovation and discovery. From its humble beginnings in the 1960s to its current applications in medicine, AR has come a long way. With its ability to enhance the real world with digital information, AR is poised to revolutionize not only medicine but also various other industries, making it an exciting field to watch for everyone interested in the potential of this technology.

Types of Augmented Reality Systems

Augmented Reality (AR) has increasingly gained attention and popularity, revolutionizing various industries, including medicine. This subchapter aims to introduce the different types of augmented reality systems used in the field of medicine. Whether you are a healthcare professional, a technology enthusiast, or simply curious about the advancements in augmented reality, this information will provide you with a comprehensive overview.

1.   Marker-based   Augmented   Reality: Marker-based AR systems utilize predefined markers or codes to overlay digital content onto the real world. These markers act as triggers, enabling the system to recognize and display the augmented reality content accurately. In medicine, markers can be used during surgical procedures to assist surgeons in visualizing internal structures, providing real-time guidance and enhancing precision.

2.   Markerless   Augmented   Reality: Unlike marker-based systems, markerless AR does not require predefined markers. Instead, it uses advanced computer vision techniques to detect and track objects or surfaces in the real world. This type of AR is particularly useful in medical education and training, where learners can interact with virtual anatomical models or simulations without the need for physical markers.

3.   Projection-based   Augmented   Reality: Projection-based AR systems project digital content directly onto real-world objects or surfaces, creating an augmented experience. In medicine, this technology can be used to project patient data, such as vital signs or medical images, onto the patient's body, allowing

healthcare professionals to access crucial information in real-time during procedures.

4.   Superimposition-based   Augmented   Reality: Superimposition-based AR combines real-time data with pre-existing images or videos. By aligning the virtual content with the real-world view, this type of AR enhances the perception of reality. In medicine, superimposition-based AR can be used to visualize medical imaging scans, such as CT or MRI, directly onto a patient's body, enabling surgeons to accurately plan and execute complex procedures.

5.   Wearable   Augmented   Reality: Wearable AR systems involve the use of head-mounted displays or smart glasses to overlay digital content onto the user's field of view. These devices provide a hands-free AR experience, making them ideal for medical professionals who require real-time information during surgeries or emergency situations. Wearable AR can also be used to provide personalized patient information, such as medical history or allergies, to healthcare providers.

In conclusion, augmented reality systems have revolutionized the field of medicine, providing innovative solutions to enhance healthcare delivery, education, and training. Whether it is marker-based, markerless, projection-based, superimposition-based, or wearable AR, each system offers unique capabilities and benefits. As augmented reality continues to evolve, its potential to revolutionize medicine and improve patient outcomes is truly remarkable.

Chapter 3: Augmented Reality in Medical Education and Training

Enhancing Medical Education with Augmented Reality

In recent years, Augmented Reality (AR) has emerged as a transformative technology, revolutionizing various industries. One field that has benefited greatly from AR is medicine. Medical education, in particular, has seen significant advancements with the integration of this innovative technology. By merging virtual elements with the real world, AR provides a unique and immersive learning experience for students and professionals alike.

Augmented Reality enables medical students to visualize complex anatomical structures and physiological processes in ways never before possible. With the use of AR devices such as smart glasses or smartphones, learners can overlay digital information onto physical objects, enhancing their understanding and retention of critical medical knowledge. For example, an anatomy class can be transformed by projecting 3D models of organs onto physical mannequins, allowing students to explore and interact with the structures in a dynamic and engaging manner.

Additionally, AR can simulate realistic medical scenarios, providing students with invaluable hands-on training without the need for live patients. This technology allows learners to practice surgical procedures, diagnose illnesses, and respond to emergencies, all within a safe and controlled virtual environment. By offering a risk-free space to make mistakes and learn from them, AR empowers aspiring medical professionals to develop their skills and confidence before entering the operating room or clinic.

Moreover, AR can facilitate collaborative learning experiences by connecting students from different locations. Through shared AR platforms, learners can interact with virtual models simultaneously, enabling real-time discussions and problem-solving. This collaborative aspect of AR not only enhances the educational experience but also fosters teamwork and communication skills, which are vital in the medical field.

Furthermore, AR can bridge the gap between theoretical knowledge and practical application. By overlaying relevant information onto real-world patient cases, AR enables medical students to analyze symptoms, interpret diagnostic tests, and make informed decisions. This integration of virtual and physical data empowers learners to develop a comprehensive understanding of medical concepts and apply them effectively in clinical settings.

In conclusion, Augmented Reality has the potential to revolutionize medical education by providing a dynamic and immersive learning experience. By enhancing visualization, simulation, collaboration, and application of medical knowledge, AR prepares aspiring medical professionals more effectively than traditional methods. As this technology continues to evolve, we can expect an even greater transformation in medical education, ultimately leading to improved patient care and outcomes. Whether you are a student, healthcare professional, or simply interested in the field of Augmented Reality, exploring the possibilities of AR in medical education is a fascinating journey that holds promise for the future of medicine.

Virtual Anatomy Simulations

In recent years, technology has made significant strides in revolutionizing various industries, and the field of medicine is no exception. Augmented Reality (AR) has emerged as a powerful tool in transforming the way doctors, medical students, and patients perceive and understand the intricacies of the human body. One of the most groundbreaking applications of AR in medicine is virtual anatomy simulations.

Virtual anatomy simulations provide an immersive and interactive experience that allows medical professionals and students to explore the human body in ways that were previously unimaginable. Using AR headsets or even mobile devices, users can visualize and manipulate three-dimensional models of organs, tissues, and skeletal structures. These simulations offer a realistic representation of the human anatomy, providing a unique opportunity to study and comprehend complex medical concepts.

For medical students, virtual anatomy simulations offer an invaluable learning experience. Traditionally, students relied on cadavers or two-dimensional illustrations to study anatomy. However, cadavers can be limited in availability, and two-dimensional images do not provide the same depth and understanding as a three-dimensional model. With virtual anatomy simulations, students can dissect virtual bodies, zoom in on specific organs, and even witness physiological processes in real-time. This hands-on approach enhances their understanding of anatomy, leading to improved diagnostic skills and surgical techniques.

Furthermore, virtual anatomy simulations also benefit experienced medical professionals. Surgeons can practice complex procedures in a risk-free environment, allowing them to refine their skills and explore new techniques. This technology reduces the need for live patients during training, minimizing potential risks and increasing patient safety. Medical professionals can also use virtual simulations to educate patients about their conditions, visually illustrating the impact of diseases on specific organs and assisting in treatment decision-making.

The integration of AR in the medical field has not only improved education and training but has also revolutionized patient care. By providing a more accurate representation of the human body, virtual anatomy simulations enable doctors to better communicate with patients. Complex medical concepts can be simplified and visualized, ensuring patients have a clearer understanding of their conditions and treatment options. This enhanced communication fosters trust and empowers patients to actively participate in their healthcare journey.

In conclusion, virtual anatomy simulations powered by augmented reality have transformed the way medical professionals learn, train, and provide care. From medical students to experienced practitioners, these simulations offer an immersive and interactive experience that deepens understanding and improves patient outcomes. As technology continues to advance, the potential for virtual anatomy simulations to revolutionize medicine is boundless.

Surgical Training and Visualization

In recent years, the world of medicine has witnessed a remarkable transformation, thanks to the groundbreaking technology of augmented reality (AR). This emerging field has revolutionized surgical training and visualization, providing a remarkable platform for medical professionals to enhance their skills and improve patient outcomes. By blending the virtual and real worlds, augmented reality has opened up new avenues for learning, practice, and precision in the medical field.

Augmented reality has transformed surgical training by providing a realistic and immersive environment for surgeons to practice their skills. In the past, surgeons could only rely on cadavers or live patients for hands-on experience, which had limitations in terms of availability and risk. With AR, surgeons can now simulate complex surgical procedures, allowing them to rehearse and refine their techniques before stepping into an operating room. This technology enables them to visualize patient anatomy in three dimensions, explore different surgical approaches, and even experience real-time feedback during the simulation. By training in a safe and controlled environment, surgeons can enhance their skills and confidence, leading to improved patient outcomes.

Furthermore, AR has revolutionized surgical visualization by offering an unprecedented level of accuracy and precision. Traditional imaging techniques like X-rays, CT scans, or MRIs provide valuable insights, but they often fall short in providing a comprehensive view of the patient's anatomy during surgery. Augmented reality overlays digital information onto the surgeon's field of view, allowing them to see vital information such as blood vessels, nerves, or tumor margins in real-time. This augmented view eliminates the need for surgeons to constantly look away at monitors or consult separate images, thereby streamlining the surgical process and reducing the risk of errors.

The impact of augmented reality in the field of surgery extends beyond the operating room. Medical students and residents can now benefit from immersive AR experiences that simulate surgical procedures, enabling them to gain invaluable knowledge and skills. Furthermore, AR technology allows surgeons to collaborate remotely, providing expert guidance and mentoring in real-time, regardless of geographical limitations. This aspect of AR not only enhances the learning experience but also improves access to specialized surgical expertise.

In conclusion, augmented reality is revolutionizing surgical training and visualization, offering a transformative platform for medical professionals to enhance their skills and improve patient outcomes. With AR, surgeons can now practice complex procedures in a safe and controlled environment, while benefiting from real-time feedback and visualization of patient anatomy. Furthermore, AR technology enables medical students and residents to gain hands-on experience and access expert guidance, fostering a new era of collaborative learning. As augmented reality continues to evolve, its impact on the medical field will undoubtedly be profound, shaping the future of surgery and medicine as a whole.

Patient Interaction and Communication

In the rapidly evolving field of medicine, technology continues to play a significant role in transforming the way healthcare professionals interact and communicate with their patients. One of the most groundbreaking advancements in recent years has been the integration of augmented reality (AR) into medical practice. This innovative technology has revolutionized patient interaction and communication, enhancing the overall healing process.

Augmented reality offers a unique and immersive experience, enabling healthcare providers to engage with their patients in ways never thought possible before. By overlaying digital information onto the real world, AR provides a visual representation of complex medical concepts, allowing patients to better understand their conditions and treatment options. This visual aid helps bridge the gap between medical jargon and patient comprehension, ensuring clearer communication and promoting shared decision-making.

For patients, the ability to see a three-dimensional rendering of their own anatomy or a simulated surgical procedure can be truly transformative. AR technology allows patients to visualize their conditions, enabling them to grasp the intricacies of their diagnosis and treatment plan. This newfound understanding empowers patients to actively participate in their own healthcare journey, leading to improved treatment adherence and better health outcomes.

Furthermore, AR offers healthcare providers novel ways to communicate vital information to patients. Through interactive digital overlays, medical professionals can explain complex procedures, potential risks, and expected outcomes in a manner that is both engaging and easily digestible. This personalized approach fosters trust and confidence between healthcare providers and patients, ultimately strengthening the therapeutic relationship.

Beyond patient education, AR also enhances communication among healthcare teams. With the ability to share real-time information and collaborate remotely, AR facilitates effective interdisciplinary communication, leading to more efficient and comprehensive patient care. This technology enables specialists from various fields to work together seamlessly, ensuring that patients receive the best possible treatment from a team of experts.

In conclusion, the integration of augmented reality into medicine has revolutionized patient interaction and communication. By providing visual representations of medical concepts, AR empowers patients to actively engage in their healthcare decisions and enhances their understanding of their conditions. Additionally, this technology improves communication among healthcare teams, fostering collaboration and ultimately improving patient outcomes. As augmented reality continues to advance, the healing power it brings to medicine will only grow stronger, benefiting patients and healthcare providers alike.

Benefits and Limitations of Augmented Reality in Medical Education

Augmented Reality (AR) has emerged as a revolutionary technology with tremendous potential in various fields, including medical education. This subchapter will delve into the benefits and limitations of utilizing AR in medical education, shedding light on how this advanced technology can transform the way medical professionals are trained and educated.

One of the most significant advantages of incorporating AR into medical education is its ability to enhance the learning experience. AR allows students and trainees to visualize complex anatomical structures and physiological processes in a three-dimensional and interactive manner. This immersive learning experience enables a deeper understanding of the human body, leading to improved retention and recall of knowledge. By overlaying virtual objects onto the real world, AR provides a unique platform for medical students to practice surgical procedures, diagnose diseases, and perform medical simulations in a safe and controlled environment. This hands-on approach fosters critical thinking and decision-making skills, preparing future healthcare professionals for real-life scenarios.

Moreover, AR has the potential to bridge the gap between theoretical knowledge and practical application. Medical students often struggle with the transition from classrooms to clinical settings. AR can play a pivotal role in this transition by allowing students to practice clinical skills in a realistic setting before treating actual patients. By providing instant feedback and guidance, AR empowers students to refine their techniques and gain confidence in their abilities. This not only ensures patient safety but also boosts the overall quality of healthcare delivery.

Despite its numerous benefits, AR also has certain limitations in the context of medical education. One such limitation is the cost associated with implementing AR technology. The development and maintenance of AR systems can be expensive, potentially limiting its accessibility for some educational institutions. Additionally, the integration of AR into existing medical curricula requires careful planning and coordination, necessitating well-trained faculty and technical support.

Another limitation of AR in medical education is the potential for information overload. The abundance of visual information presented through AR can overwhelm students, leading to cognitive overload and reduced learning outcomes. Therefore, it is crucial to strike a balance between the amount of information provided and the student's cognitive capacity.

In conclusion, augmented reality holds immense potential in revolutionizing medical education. It offers a range of benefits, including enhanced learning experiences and improved practical skills. However, limitations such as cost and information overload must be considered when integrating AR into medical curricula. By addressing these limitations and capitalizing on its advantages, AR has the power to reshape medical education and ultimately improve patient care.

Chapter 4: Augmented Reality in Diagnosis and Treatment

Augmented Reality for Diagnostic Imaging

In recent years, Augmented Reality (AR) has emerged as a groundbreaking technology that has the potential to revolutionize the field of medicine. The integration of AR into diagnostic imaging techniques holds immense promise in enhancing the accuracy, efficiency, and overall patient experience in medical imaging.

Diagnostic imaging plays a crucial role in healthcare, aiding in the detection, diagnosis, and monitoring of various medical conditions. However, traditional imaging methods can sometimes present challenges such as limited visibility, complex interpretation, and a lack of real-time feedback. This is where AR steps in, bridging the gap between the physical world and virtual information, to provide healthcare professionals with unprecedented insights and capabilities.

By utilizing AR, medical imaging can be transformed into an interactive, immersive experience. Imagine a surgeon being able to visualize a patient's internal organs and structures in real-time during a complex procedure, overlaying vital information such as blood flow, nerve pathways, and tumor locations directly onto the patient's body. This augmented view allows for more precise and informed decision-making, leading to improved outcomes for patients.

Moreover, AR can greatly enhance the communication between healthcare professionals and patients. By overlaying diagnostic images onto the patient's body, physicians can effectively explain medical conditions, treatment options, and potential outcomes in a more understandable and engaging manner. This not only empowers patients to take an active role in their healthcare journey but also fosters a stronger doctor-patient relationship.

Furthermore, AR can streamline the diagnostic process by providing real-time feedback and guidance to radiologists and other healthcare professionals. By integrating AR into imaging devices, radiologists can navigate through complex datasets with ease, highlighting areas of concern, and improving the accuracy of their diagnoses. This technology also has the potential to reduce the need for repeat scans and invasive procedures, minimizing patient discomfort and healthcare costs.

While the potential of AR for diagnostic imaging is vast, it is important to address the challenges and ethical considerations that come with its implementation. Ensuring patient privacy, data security, and proper training for healthcare professionals are essential in harnessing the full potential of this technology.

In conclusion, Augmented Reality has the power to revolutionize diagnostic imaging, offering healthcare professionals a new level of insight, precision, and collaboration. By integrating AR into medical imaging techniques, we can expect improved diagnosis accuracy, enhanced patient communication, and more efficient healthcare delivery. As this technology continues to evolve, it is crucial for the medical community to embrace and harness its capabilities for the betterment of patient care and outcomes.

Overlaying Medical Images onto Patients

In recent years, the field of Augmented Reality (AR) has made tremendous advancements, revolutionizing various industries, including medicine. AR has the potential to transform the way medical professionals diagnose and treat patients, opening up new possibilities for improved healthcare outcomes. One of the most exciting applications of AR in medicine is the ability to overlay medical images onto patients, providing physicians with a real-time, interactive visualization of the patient's anatomy.

Imagine a surgeon preparing for a complex procedure. Traditionally, they would rely on static images or two-dimensional scans to guide them. However, with the integration of AR technology, these images can be overlayed directly onto the patient's body, providing a three-dimensional representation of the affected area. This allows the surgeon to see the internal structures in real-time, enhancing their ability to navigate through complex anatomical regions.

The benefits of overlaying medical images onto patients are not limited to surgical interventions alone. In the field of radiology, AR technology can be utilized to provide radiologists with an enhanced understanding of a patient's condition. By overlaying medical images onto the patient, radiologists can precisely locate abnormalities, such as tumors or lesions, and gain a better understanding of their size, shape, and proximity to surrounding structures. This information is invaluable when developing treatment plans or monitoring the progress of a disease.

Furthermore, AR has the potential to improve patient education and engagement. By overlaying medical images onto their own bodies, patients can have a better visual understanding of their condition. This empowers them to actively participate in their healthcare decisions, as they can see firsthand the areas affected and the proposed treatments. Additionally, medical professionals can use AR technology to explain complex procedures or anatomical concepts to patients, simplifying the communication process and increasing patient satisfaction.

While the integration of AR in medicine is still in its early stages, the potential for improving patient care is vast. As this technology continues to evolve, we can expect to see more advanced AR systems capable of providing real-time, interactive overlays of medical images onto patients. This will undoubtedly transform the way healthcare professionals diagnose, treat, and communicate with their patients.

In conclusion, the overlaying of medical images onto patients through AR technology represents a significant advancement in the field of medicine. It has the potential to enhance surgical precision, aid in radiological diagnosis, and improve patient education and engagement. As this technology continues to develop, the healing power of augmented reality will undoubtedly revolutionize medicine, benefiting both medical professionals and patients alike.

Guided Biopsies and Interventions

Guided Biopsies and Interventions: Revolutionizing Medicine with Augmented Reality

Augmented Reality (AR) is rapidly transforming the field of medicine, offering innovative solutions to enhance diagnostic and interventional procedures. One groundbreaking application of AR in healthcare is in the realm of guided biopsies and interventions. This technology is revolutionizing the way physicians perform these procedures, providing greater precision, efficiency, and patient safety.

Traditionally, biopsies and interventions have relied on the expertise of physicians and the use of medical imaging technologies such as ultrasound, MRI, or CT scans. While these imaging techniques provide valuable information, they often require physicians to mentally integrate the two-dimensional images with the three-dimensional anatomy of the patient. This can lead to human errors, longer procedure times, and potential complications.

With the integration of AR, physicians can now visualize and interact with virtual anatomical structures overlaid onto the patient's body in real-time. This enables them to precisely target the area of interest, reducing the risk of sampling errors and improving diagnostic accuracy. By superimposing virtual images onto the patient's body, AR provides a natural and intuitive way for physicians to navigate through complex anatomical structures during biopsies and interventions.

Furthermore, AR-guided biopsies and interventions also offer significant benefits to patients. By eliminating the need for multiple imaging scans and reducing procedure times, patients experience less discomfort and stress. AR technology also allows for better patient education, as physicians can use visual cues and interactive models to explain the procedure and expected outcomes. This empowers patients to make informed decisions about their healthcare and improves their overall satisfaction with the treatment process.

The potential applications of AR in guided biopsies and interventions are vast. From the precise targeting of tumors during cancer biopsies to the guidance of surgical instruments during minimally invasive procedures, AR is transforming the way healthcare professionals approach these critical interventions. As the technology continues to advance, we can expect even more sophisticated AR tools that will further enhance procedural accuracy and patient outcomes.

In conclusion, guided biopsies and interventions augmented by AR are revolutionizing medicine. This technology is empowering physicians to perform procedures with greater precision and efficiency, while also improving patient safety and satisfaction. The integration of AR into healthcare is not only transforming the way physicians navigate through complex anatomical structures but also enhancing patient education and decision-making. As the field of augmented reality continues to evolve, the future of guided biopsies and interventions looks promising, holding immense potential for the advancement of medicine as a whole.

Augmented Reality-assisted Surgeries

In recent years, the field of medicine has witnessed remarkable advancements. One such breakthrough is the integration of augmented reality (AR) technology into surgical procedures, revolutionizing the way surgeries are performed and enhancing patient outcomes. This subchapter explores the fascinating world of augmented reality-assisted surgeries and how this technology is reshaping the future of medicine.

Augmented reality, a technology that overlays virtual information onto the real world, has found its way into various industries, and healthcare is no exception. By superimposing digital images, videos, and 3D models onto the surgeon's field of vision, AR-assisted surgeries offer a wealth of benefits. Surgeons can now visualize complex anatomical structures, identify vital organs, and precisely navigate through intricate surgical pathways.

One of the most significant advantages of AR-assisted surgeries is the increased accuracy and precision it offers. Surgeons can now perform complex procedures with unprecedented accuracy, minimizing the risk of errors and complications. AR technology provides real-time feedback, allowing surgeons to make informed decisions and adjust their actions accordingly.

Furthermore, AR-assisted surgeries improve surgical education and training. Medical students and aspiring surgeons can now gain valuable hands-on experience in a virtual environment, practicing complex procedures repeatedly until they achieve mastery. This immersive training significantly reduces the learning curve, ensuring that surgeons are well-prepared and confident when performing actual surgeries.

Patient outcomes are also greatly improved with AR-assisted surgeries. The enhanced visualization capabilities of AR enable surgeons to perform minimally invasive procedures with greater efficacy. This results in smaller incisions, reduced scarring, and faster recovery times for patients. In addition, AR technology allows surgeons to personalize treatments, tailoring surgical plans to the specific needs of each patient.

While the field of AR-assisted surgeries is still relatively new, the potential for growth and innovation is immense. As technology continues to advance, we can anticipate even more sophisticated augmented reality tools, such as haptic feedback systems and real-time data integration, further enhancing surgical precision and patient safety.

In conclusion, augmented reality-assisted surgeries represent a significant milestone in medical innovation. This technology has the potential to transform the way surgeries are performed, improving patient outcomes, and reducing risks. As the field continues to evolve, it is crucial for healthcare professionals and researchers to embrace and explore the possibilities offered by augmented reality, ultimately revolutionizing the practice of medicine for the better.

Navigation and Precision in Surgical Procedures

In recent years, the field of medicine has witnessed remarkable advancements that have revolutionized the way surgical procedures are performed. One such groundbreaking technology is augmented reality (AR), which has the potential to enhance navigation and precision during surgical interventions. This subchapter delves into the incredible possibilities that AR brings to the operating room, addressing the audience of "everyone" and specifically targeting those interested in the niche of augmented reality.

Augmented reality technology integrates computer-generated information into the real-world environment, providing surgeons with enhanced visualization and guidance during surgical procedures. By superimposing digital images onto the surgeon's view, AR enables them to navigate complex anatomical structures with greater accuracy and confidence. This technology has the ability to transform surgery into a more precise and efficient process, ultimately leading to improved patient outcomes.

One of the key advantages of AR in surgical procedures is its ability to provide real-time feedback to the surgeon. By overlaying critical information such as anatomical landmarks, vital signs, and preoperative images onto the surgical field, AR allows the surgeon to make more informed decisions during the operation. This real-time feedback helps reduce the margin of error and enhances the overall safety of the surgical procedure.

Furthermore, AR facilitates surgical planning and simulation. Surgeons can use AR to preoperatively map out the surgical site, enabling them to visualize the procedure and identify potential challenges. This preoperative planning allows for more precise surgical techniques, reducing the risk of complications and improving patient outcomes. Moreover, AR can simulate the procedure in a virtual environment, allowing surgeons to practice complex maneuvers and enhance their skills before entering the operating room.

Augmented reality also has the potential to improve surgical training and education. By providing a virtual environment that replicates real surgical scenarios, AR allows trainees to gain hands-on experience and develop their skills in a safe and controlled setting. This technology can accelerate the learning curve for aspiring surgeons and foster a new generation of highly skilled professionals.

In conclusion, the integration of augmented reality into surgical procedures holds immense potential for navigation and precision. By providing real-time feedback, facilitating surgical planning, and enhancing training opportunities, AR promises to revolutionize the field of medicine. As this technology continues to evolve, it is essential for healthcare professionals and the general public to stay informed and embrace the transformative power of augmented reality in medicine.

Real-time Visualization of Patient Data

In the ever-evolving field of medicine, the integration of augmented reality (AR) has brought forth a new era of possibilities. One of the most groundbreaking applications of AR in healthcare is its ability to provide real-time visualization of patient data. This subchapter aims to delve into the incredible impact that AR has had on the visualization of patient data, revolutionizing the way healthcare professionals understand, analyze, and interpret vital information.

Augmented reality technology allows healthcare providers to overlay patient data onto the physical world, enabling them to see and interact with information in real time. By wearing AR devices such as smart glasses or using AR-enabled mobile applications, doctors, nurses, and other medical personnel can seamlessly access and visualize patient data directly in their field of view. This not only eliminates the need to constantly refer to traditional computer screens or medical records but also enhances decision-making processes and improves patient outcomes.

The real-time visualization of patient data through augmented reality offers numerous advantages. Firstly, it enables healthcare professionals to have immediate access to critical information, such as vital signs, medical history, lab results, and medication records. This accessibility allows for quicker and more accurate diagnoses, especially during emergency situations where time plays a crucial role.

Furthermore, AR visualization enhances medical education and training. Students and aspiring healthcare professionals can learn complex concepts more effectively by visualizing patient data in real-time scenarios. They can practice diagnosing and treating virtual patients, gaining hands-on experience without compromising the safety and well-being of real patients.

Additionally, real-time visualization of patient data through AR facilitates remote collaboration among healthcare professionals. Specialists from different locations can virtually come together, review patient information, and provide consultations in real time. This not only improves the quality of care but also reduces costs and enhances access to specialized expertise, particularly in underserved areas.

While the potential of real-time visualization of patient data through augmented reality is immense, it is crucial to address concerns regarding data privacy and security. Striking a balance between reaping the benefits of AR technology and safeguarding sensitive patient information is of utmost importance.

In conclusion, the advent of augmented reality has unlocked a world of possibilities in healthcare, particularly in the visualization of patient data. By providing real-time access to critical information, AR empowers healthcare professionals to make better-informed decisions, improves medical education, and fosters remote collaboration among specialists. As this technology continues to evolve, the healing power of augmented reality is poised to revolutionize medicine for the betterment of everyone.

Rehabilitation and Physical Therapy with Augmented Reality

In recent years, the field of healthcare has witnessed a remarkable transformation with the integration of augmented reality (AR). Augmented reality refers to the technology that superimposes digital content onto the real world, enhancing our perception and interaction with the environment. This groundbreaking technology has opened up new possibilities in various medical specialties, including rehabilitation and physical therapy.

Rehabilitation is a crucial aspect of healthcare, aiding individuals in recovering from injuries, surgeries, or disabilities. Traditionally, physical therapy has relied on manual exercises and techniques to restore movement and function. However, with the advent of augmented reality, the rehabilitation process has been revolutionized, providing patients with innovative and engaging therapy experiences.

One of the key benefits of augmented reality in rehabilitation is its ability to create immersive and interactive environments. By wearing AR headsets or using mobile devices, patients can engage in virtual scenarios that simulate real-life situations. For instance, a patient recovering from a stroke can use AR to practice daily activities such as cooking or dressing in a safe and controlled environment. This not only helps in regaining motor skills but also boosts confidence and independence.

Furthermore, augmented reality enables therapists to monitor and analyze patients' progress more effectively. With AR devices, therapists can track joint movements, muscle strength, and range of motion in real-time. This data can be analyzed to tailor personalized treatment plans and make adjustments accordingly. Additionally, therapists can provide immediate feedback and guidance during therapy sessions, enhancing the overall quality of care.

Augmented reality also offers gamification elements to rehabilitation, making therapy sessions more enjoyable and motivating for patients. By integrating game-like features and challenges, AR-based exercises encourage active participation and long-term engagement. Patients can compete with themselves or others, unlocking achievements and rewards along the way. The element of fun and competition not only improves adherence to therapy but also stimulates neural plasticity, accelerating recovery.

In conclusion, augmented reality has transformed the field of rehabilitation and physical therapy, offering innovative solutions that enhance patient outcomes. By creating immersive environments, monitoring progress, and incorporating gamification elements, AR has revolutionized the therapy experience. This technology holds immense potential for improving the quality of care and expanding access to rehabilitation services. As augmented reality continues to evolve, its integration in healthcare will undoubtedly shape the future of medicine, benefiting patients of all ages and conditions.

Chapter 5: Ethical and Legal Considerations of Augmented Reality in Medicine

Privacy and Data Security Concerns

In recent years, the rapid advancement of technology has brought about numerous innovations, and one of the most groundbreaking is augmented reality (AR). Augmented reality has the potential to revolutionize the field of medicine, providing doctors and healthcare professionals with new tools and techniques to enhance patient care and treatment outcomes. However, along with these exciting prospects, there are also concerns surrounding privacy and data security that need to be addressed.

Augmented reality in medicine involves the use of computer-generated sensory inputs, such as graphics, sound, and haptic feedback, to enhance the real-world environment. This fusion of virtual and real elements has proven to be immensely beneficial in various medical applications, including surgical simulations, medical training, and patient education. However, as the use of AR in healthcare becomes more prevalent, it is crucial to consider the potential privacy risks and data security vulnerabilities that may arise.

One of the primary concerns surrounding AR in medicine is the collection and storage of personal health data. As augmented reality devices and applications become increasingly integrated into the healthcare system, they have the ability to gather a vast amount of sensitive information about patients. This data can include medical records, diagnostic results, and even real-time physiological data. It is essential to establish robust privacy protocols and data protection measures to ensure that this information remains secure and confidential.

Another area of concern is the potential for unauthorized access to AR systems. As augmented reality devices become more interconnected and reliant on networks, they become susceptible to hacking and cyberattacks. A breach in the security of an AR system could lead to unauthorized access to patient data, manipulation of medical images or information, and even disruption of critical medical procedures. It is imperative for healthcare organizations and technology developers to implement stringent security measures to safeguard against these threats.

Additionally, there is a need to address the ethical implications of augmented reality in healthcare. With the ability to overlay virtual information onto the real world, there is a potential for misuse or inappropriate sharing of patient data. It is crucial to establish clear guidelines and regulations to ensure the responsible and ethical use of AR technology in the medical field.

In conclusion, while augmented reality holds tremendous potential to revolutionize medicine, it is essential to address the privacy and data security concerns associated with its use. Robust privacy protocols, data protection measures, and stringent security measures must be implemented to safeguard patient information and prevent unauthorized access. Furthermore, ethical considerations should guide the responsible use of AR technology to ensure patient privacy and trust in the healthcare system. By addressing these concerns head-on, we can fully harness the healing power of augmented reality while protecting individual privacy and data security.

Regulatory and Compliance Issues

In the rapidly evolving field of augmented reality (AR), where technology is revolutionizing the medical industry, it is essential to be aware of the regulatory and compliance issues surrounding this innovative technology. As AR becomes more prevalent in healthcare, it is crucial for both professionals and users to understand the potential risks, challenges, and legal considerations that come with its implementation.

One of the primary concerns in the regulatory landscape of AR is patient privacy. With the integration of AR in medical procedures, the collection and storage of patient data become more prevalent. Adhering to strict privacy regulations, such as the Health Insurance Portability and Accountability Act (HIPAA), is essential to safeguard patient information and maintain their trust in the healthcare system. Medical practitioners and developers must ensure that AR applications comply with these regulations and implement measures to protect patient confidentiality.

Another significant aspect of regulatory compliance in AR is the approval process for medical devices or applications. As AR technology is increasingly used in diagnostic and therapeutic procedures, it falls under the purview of regulatory bodies, such as the Food and Drug Administration (FDA). Developers must navigate the complex regulatory landscape to obtain the necessary approvals and certifications for their AR applications to ensure patient safety and efficacy.

Additionally, issues related to liability and malpractice may arise in the context of augmented reality. Healthcare professionals must understand their responsibilities and potential risks when using AR in patient care. It is crucial to establish clear guidelines and protocols to minimize the chances of errors or misdiagnoses due to the use of AR technology. Ensuring adequate training and education for healthcare providers using AR is vital to prevent any legal or ethical implications.

Moreover, as AR continues to advance, ethical considerations must be taken into account. For instance, augmented reality can blur the lines between reality and virtual experiences, potentially leading to psychological or emotional harm to users. It is important to establish ethical guidelines and standards to prevent the misuse or abuse of AR technology in medical settings.

In conclusion, as augmented reality gains prominence in the medical field, understanding the regulatory and compliance issues associated with this technology is paramount. Patient privacy, regulatory approvals, liability, and ethical considerations are crucial aspects that need to be addressed to ensure the safe and responsible use of AR in healthcare. By staying informed and adhering to the appropriate regulations, we can fully harness the healing power of augmented reality while maintaining the highest standards of care and compliance.

Informed Consent and Patient Autonomy

Informed Consent and Patient Autonomy: Empowering Healthcare through Augmented Reality

In the rapidly advancing field of healthcare, the integration of augmented reality (AR) technology has revolutionized the way medical professionals engage with patients. This subchapter delves into the crucial topics of informed consent and patient autonomy, highlighting the transformative potential of AR in empowering individuals and enhancing their healthcare experiences.

Informed consent, a fundamental ethical principle in medicine, ensures that patients have a comprehensive understanding of their medical condition, treatment options, potential risks, and benefits before making informed decisions about their care. Augmented reality has emerged as a powerful tool in facilitating this process, as it enables healthcare providers to present complex medical information in a visually immersive and easily understandable manner.

By overlaying digital information onto the real world, AR empowers patients to actively participate in their treatment plans through enhanced visualization and interaction. For instance, imagine a patient diagnosed with a heart condition, who can now don a pair of AR glasses to see a detailed 3D representation of their heart. This augmented visualization not only helps patients grasp the intricacies of their condition but also fosters a deeper sense of engagement and ownership over their healthcare journey.

Moreover, AR technology allows patients to explore various treatment options virtually, experiencing simulations of potential outcomes and side effects. This experiential understanding of different interventions empowers patients to make well-informed decisions, promoting patient autonomy and ensuring their preferences are respected throughout the treatment process.

Informed consent is not just limited to medical procedures; it also extends to clinical trials and research studies. AR can play a pivotal role in this context as well. By providing participants with immersive simulations of the trial process, potential risks, and anticipated benefits, AR promotes transparency and supports individuals in making informed decisions about their participation.

Furthermore, augmented reality can be utilized as a powerful educational tool for patients, delivering personalized information and self-management strategies directly to their fingertips. Through AR-enabled smartphone applications or wearable devices, patients can access real-time data, reminders, and instructional videos, empowering them to actively engage in their own care, manage chronic conditions, and make healthier lifestyle choices.

In conclusion, augmented reality has the potential to revolutionize the healthcare landscape by promoting informed consent and patient autonomy. By enhancing visualization, facilitating virtual simulations, and providing personalized educational resources, AR empowers individuals to actively participate in their healthcare decisions and take ownership of their well-being. As the integration of augmented reality technology continues to advance, the future of medicine holds immense promise for transforming healthcare into a truly patient-centered and empowering experience for everyone.

Potential Impact on Healthcare Providers and Workforce

The rapid advancements in technology, particularly in the field of augmented reality (AR), are revolutionizing the healthcare industry. Augmented reality has the potential to transform the way healthcare providers deliver medical care and the overall workforce dynamics in the industry. This subchapter aims to explore the potential impact of AR on healthcare providers and the workforce as a whole.

One of the significant benefits of AR in healthcare is the enhanced training and education it offers to healthcare providers. With AR, medical students and professionals can have access to realistic simulations and virtual anatomical models, allowing for more immersive learning experiences. This technology enables healthcare providers to practice complex procedures in a safe and controlled environment, reducing the risk of errors during actual patient care. As a result, AR can significantly improve the competence and confidence of healthcare professionals, ultimately leading to better patient outcomes.

Moreover, AR can streamline and improve the efficiency of healthcare workflows. By overlaying digital information onto the real-world environment, AR can assist healthcare providers in accessing patient information, vital signs, and medical records in real-time. This instant access to critical data can save valuable time, reduce the risk of medical errors, and enhance the overall quality of care. Additionally, AR can provide real-time guidance during surgical procedures, aiding surgeons in precise navigation and visualization, leading to improved surgical outcomes.

The introduction of AR technology in healthcare may also reshape the workforce dynamics. The demand for skilled AR developers, designers, and technicians will likely increase as the industry embraces this transformative technology. This will create new job opportunities and career paths for individuals with a background in augmented reality. Moreover, healthcare providers will need to adapt to the use of AR and undergo training to effectively utilize this technology. This shift in the workforce will require a collaborative effort between technology experts and healthcare professionals to ensure a smooth integration of AR into healthcare settings.

In conclusion, the potential impact of augmented reality on healthcare providers and the workforce is immense. From improved training and education to streamlined workflows and new job opportunities, AR has the power to revolutionize the healthcare industry. As this technology continues to evolve, it is crucial for healthcare professionals, technology experts, and policymakers to collaborate and embrace the possibilities that augmented reality offers. By harnessing the healing power of augmented reality, we can usher in a new era of medicine that is more efficient, precise, and patient-centered.

Chapter 6: Future Perspectives and Challenges

Advancements in Augmented Reality Technology

Augmented Reality (AR) has come a long way since its inception, and the field is constantly evolving with groundbreaking advancements. This subchapter explores some of the most exciting developments in AR technology, focusing on how they are revolutionizing various industries and improving our everyday lives. Whether you are an AR enthusiast or simply curious about the latest technological advancements, this section will provide you with a comprehensive overview.

One of the most significant advancements in AR technology is the development of wearable devices. These devices, such as smart glasses and headsets, allow users to experience augmented reality in a hands-free and immersive way. With the ability to overlay digital information onto the real world, these devices have transformed industries like healthcare, education, and manufacturing. Surgeons can now perform complex procedures with real-time guidance and visualizations, while students can learn through interactive and engaging AR experiences.

Another key advancement in AR technology is the improvement in tracking and sensing capabilities. With advancements in computer vision and sensor technologies, AR systems can now accurately recognize and track objects in the real world. This enables precise placement and interaction of virtual objects, enhancing the user's experience. From gaming to interior design, this technology has opened up new possibilities for creative expression and problem-solving.

Furthermore, the integration of Artificial Intelligence (AI) has propelled AR technology to new heights. AI algorithms can analyze vast amounts of data and provide real-time insights, making AR applications more intelligent and responsive. For example, AR-powered medical devices can quickly analyze patient data and provide doctors with valuable information during diagnosis and treatment. In the retail industry, AI-powered AR applications can personalize shopping experiences by offering tailored product recommendations based on individual preferences.

Advancements in AR technology have also led to the emergence of social AR experiences. With the introduction of AR filters and effects on social media platforms, users can now share interactive and immersive content with their friends and followers. This has transformed the way we communicate and express ourselves online, fostering a sense of community and creativity.

In conclusion, the advancements in augmented reality technology have revolutionized various industries and improved our daily lives. From wearable devices to improved tracking capabilities and the integration of AI, AR has become more accessible, intelligent, and immersive. The potential applications of this technology are vast, and its impact on society will continue to grow. As AR continues to evolve, we can expect even more exciting advancements that will shape the way we perceive and interact with the world around us.

Integrating Augmented Reality into the Healthcare System

Augmented Reality (AR) has emerged as a groundbreaking technology that has the potential to revolutionize various industries, and the healthcare sector is no exception. With its ability to overlay digital information onto the real world, AR holds immense promise in enhancing medical practices, improving patient outcomes, and transforming the way healthcare professionals work. This subchapter explores the exciting possibilities of integrating Augmented Reality into the healthcare system and how it is poised to reshape the future of medicine.

One of the most significant applications of AR in healthcare is in surgical procedures. Surgeons can utilize AR to overlay real-time patient data, such as medical imaging scans, directly onto their field of view during an operation. This allows for a more precise and efficient surgery, as surgeons can visualize critical anatomical structures without having to look away from the patient. AR also enables surgeons to access real-time guidance and instructions, reducing the risk of errors and improving surgical outcomes.

Moreover, AR can revolutionize medical training and education. With AR, medical students and professionals can immerse themselves in realistic virtual environments that simulate various medical conditions and procedures. This technology enables them to gain hands-on experience, practice complex surgeries, and enhance their diagnostic skills in a safe and controlled setting. AR also has the potential to democratize medical education by providing accessible and cost-effective training solutions to healthcare providers worldwide.

In addition to surgical applications, AR can improve patient care and engagement. By using AR-enabled devices, patients can access personalized information about their conditions, medications, and treatment plans in real-time. This empowers patients to take an active role in their own healthcare journey and make informed decisions. AR can also be used to provide visualizations of complex medical concepts, helping patients better understand their diagnoses and treatment options.

Furthermore, AR can assist in remote healthcare delivery, enabling healthcare professionals to provide virtual consultations and monitor patients from a distance. This is particularly beneficial for individuals who live in remote areas or have limited access to medical facilities. Through AR, doctors can virtually examine patients, offer medical advice, and remotely monitor their vital signs, ensuring timely and efficient healthcare delivery.

In conclusion, integrating Augmented Reality into the healthcare system holds tremendous potential for improving medical practices, enhancing patient care, and transforming the way healthcare professionals work. From surgical procedures and medical training to patient engagement and remote healthcare delivery, AR is poised to revolutionize medicine. As this technology continues to evolve, it is imperative for healthcare professionals and stakeholders to embrace AR's capabilities and harness its power to shape a more efficient, accessible, and patient-centered healthcare system.

Overcoming Barriers to Implementation

Introduction:

In the realm of augmented reality (AR), the potential for revolutionizing medicine is immense. The integration of virtual elements into the real world opens doors to enhanced diagnosis, treatment, and patient care. However, despite the numerous benefits, there are several barriers that need to be addressed to ensure the successful implementation of AR technology in healthcare settings. In this subchapter, we will explore these barriers and discuss strategies for overcoming them.

1.   Technological   Challenges:
One significant barrier to implementing AR in medicine is the technological hurdles associated with developing and maintaining the required infrastructure. AR systems demand sophisticated hardware, software, and network connectivity. Additionally, ensuring compatibility across different devices and platforms can be challenging. By investing in research and development, collaborating with technology companies, and promoting interoperability standards, these hurdles can be overcome.

2.   Cost   Considerations:
Cost is another barrier that hinders the widespread adoption of AR in medicine. The expenses associated with developing, acquiring, and maintaining AR systems may pose challenges for healthcare organizations, particularly smaller ones. Collaborations between healthcare providers, technology companies, and governments can help alleviate this barrier by providing financial support, grants, or tax incentives for AR implementation.

3.			Training			and			Education: Healthcare professionals often lack the necessary training and education to effectively utilize AR technology. Overcoming this barrier requires comprehensive training programs that equip healthcare workers with the knowledge and skills needed to leverage AR tools. Incorporating AR training modules into medical school curricula and providing continuous professional development opportunities will ensure that healthcare professionals are proficient in using AR for diagnostics, surgery, and patient care.

4.			Legal			and			Ethical			Concerns: The implementation of AR in medicine raises legal and ethical questions that must be addressed. Issues related to patient privacy, data security, and liability need to be carefully considered and regulated. Collaborations between healthcare professionals, technology experts, and legal authorities can help establish guidelines and regulations that protect patient rights while enabling the seamless integration of AR technology into medical practice.

5.			Acceptance			and			Cultural			Shift: Lastly, overcoming the barrier of acceptance and cultural shift is crucial for successful AR implementation. Resistance to change, skepticism, and fear of technology can hinder progress. Educating and involving stakeholders, such as patients, healthcare providers, and policymakers, in the benefits of AR technology will foster acceptance and promote a cultural shift towards embracing AR in healthcare.

Conclusion:
Overcoming barriers to implementing AR in medicine requires a multi-faceted approach that addresses technological challenges, cost considerations, training and education needs, legal and ethical

concerns, and acceptance and cultural shift. By actively working towards overcoming these barriers, we can unlock the full potential of augmented reality and revolutionize medicine, ultimately improving patient outcomes and transforming healthcare for everyone.

Implications for Medical Research and Innovation

As the field of augmented reality continues to evolve and make remarkable strides in various industries, one area where its potential truly shines is in the field of medicine. Augmented reality has opened up a whole new world of possibilities for medical research and innovation, revolutionizing the way we approach and practice medicine. In this subchapter, we will explore the implications of augmented reality in medical research and innovation and the profound impact it can have on healthcare.

One of the most significant implications of augmented reality in medical research is its ability to enhance the visualization and understanding of complex anatomical structures. Through the use of AR devices, medical professionals can now view three-dimensional representations of organs, tissues, and even microscopic structures in real-time. This level of detail and accuracy provides researchers with invaluable insights into the human body, enabling them to better understand diseases, develop targeted treatment plans, and improve surgical procedures.

Additionally, augmented reality can revolutionize medical education and training. Traditionally, medical students rely on textbooks, lectures, and limited hands-on experiences to learn complex procedures and techniques. However, with AR, students can now engage in immersive and interactive learning experiences. They can practice surgeries, simulate patient encounters, and gain practical skills in a safe and controlled environment. This not only enhances their understanding but also improves patient outcomes as doctors are better trained and prepared.

Furthermore, augmented reality has the potential to transform patient care and improve clinical outcomes. By overlaying digital information onto the real world, doctors can access patient data, medical records, and diagnostic imaging in real-time. This allows for more efficient and accurate diagnoses, personalized treatment plans, and improved patient-doctor communication. Additionally, AR can aid in remote patient monitoring, enabling healthcare professionals to remotely assess patients and provide timely interventions, especially in areas with limited access to specialized medical care.

In conclusion, the implications of augmented reality in medical research and innovation are vast and game-changing. From enhancing visualization and understanding of complex anatomical structures to revolutionizing medical education and training, and even transforming patient care and clinical outcomes, AR has the potential to revolutionize the field of medicine. With continued advancements in technology and increased adoption of augmented reality in healthcare, we can expect to witness groundbreaking discoveries, improved treatment options, and ultimately, a revolutionized healthcare system for the betterment of all.

Chapter 7: Conclusion

Recap of Key Points

In this subchapter, we will summarize the key points discussed throughout the book "The Healing Power of Augmented Reality: Revolutionizing Medicine." This recap is designed to help everyone, including those interested in the field of Augmented Reality, gain a comprehensive understanding of the book's main ideas.

Augmented Reality (AR) refers to the technology that enhances our real-world environment by overlaying digital information, such as images, videos, or sounds, onto it. This revolutionary technology has immense potential in the field of medicine, transforming the way we diagnose, treat, and manage various medical conditions.

One of the crucial points highlighted in this book is the ability of AR to improve medical education and training. By utilizing AR, medical students and professionals can gain a more immersive and interactive learning experience. AR simulations allow them to practice complex procedures in a safe and controlled environment, enhancing their skills and confidence.

Another significant aspect of AR in medicine is its contribution to surgical interventions. Surgeons can now use AR-assisted navigation systems that project critical information, such as patient data, anatomical structures, and surgical plans, directly onto their field of view. This real-time guidance improves precision, reduces errors, and ultimately leads to better patient outcomes.

Additionally, AR has the potential to revolutionize telemedicine and remote patient care. With the help of AR devices, healthcare providers can remotely assess patients, visualize symptoms, and guide them through self-diagnosis or treatment procedures. This technology has the potential to bridge geographical barriers and provide medical assistance to individuals in remote or underserved areas.

Furthermore, the book emphasizes the importance of user experience and design in AR applications. Developers need to prioritize creating intuitive and user-friendly interfaces to ensure seamless integration of AR into medical practices. This includes considering factors such as ergonomics, data visualization, and user feedback to maximize the benefits of AR in healthcare.

In conclusion, "The Healing Power of Augmented Reality: Revolutionizing Medicine" highlights the transformative potential of AR in the field of medicine. From enhancing medical education and training to improving surgical interventions and enabling remote patient care, AR is set to revolutionize healthcare as we know it. By embracing this technology and addressing the challenges associated with its implementation, we can unlock its full healing power and positively impact the lives of patients worldwide.

9 798869 045782